The Complete Diabetic Cookbook

sy Diabetic Meal Prep 2021.
on in blood sugar and reverse
Simple and healthy recipes
aring diabetic meals for
beginners.

Additionally, the information in the following pages is intended only for informational purposes and should thus be thought of as universal. As befitting its nature, it is presented without assurance regarding its prolonged validity or interim quality. Trademarks that are mentioned are done without written consent and can in no way be considered an endorsement from the trademark holder.

TABLE OF CONTENTS

BREAKFAST RECIPES

Healthy Cottage Cheese Pancakes

Preparation Time: 10 minutes

Cooking Time: 15

Servings: 1

Ingredients:

- 1/2 cup of Cottage cheese (low-fat)

- 1/3 cup (approx. 2 egg whites) Egg whites

- ¼ cup of Oats

- 1 teaspoon of Vanilla extract

- Olive oil cooking spray

- 1 tablespoon of Stevia (raw)

- Berries or sugar-free jam (optional)

Directions:

1. Begin by taking a food blender and adding in the egg whites and cottage cheese. Also add in the vanilla extract, a pinch of stevia, and oats. Palpitate until the consistency is well smooth.

2. Get a nonstick pan and oil it nicely with the cooking spray. Position the pan on low heat.

3. After it has been heated, scoop out half of the batter and pour it on the pan. Cook for about 21/2 minutes on each side.

4. Position the cooked pancakes on a serving plate and cover with sugar-free jam or berries.

Nutrition: Calories: 205 calories per serving Fat – 1.5 g, Protein – 24.5 g, Carbohydrates – 19 g

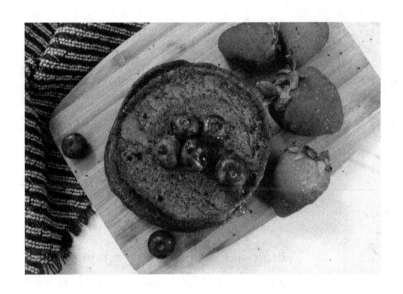

Avocado Lemon Toast

Preparation Time: 10 minutes

Cooking Time: 13 minutes

Servings: 2

Ingredients:

- Whole-grain bread – 2 slices

- Fresh cilantro (chopped) – 2 tablespoons

- Lemon zest – ¼ teaspoon

- Fine sea salt – 1 pinch

Directions:

1. Begin by getting a medium-sized mixing bowl and adding in the avocado. Make use of a fork to crush it properly.

2. Then, add in the cilantro, lemon zest, lemon juice, sea salt, and cayenne pepper. Mix well until combined.

3. Toast the bread slices in a toaster until golden brown. It should take about 3 minutes.

4. Top the toasted bread slices with the avocado mixture and finalize by drizzling with chia seeds.

Nutrition: Calories: 72 calories per serving Protein – 3.6 g Fat – 1.2 g Carbohydrates – 11.6 g

Healthy Baked Eggs

Preparation Time: 10 minutes

Cooking Time: 1 hour

Servings: 6

Ingredients:

- Olive oil – 1 tablespoon

- Garlic – 2 cloves

- Eggs – 8 larges

- Sea salt – 1/2 teaspoon

- Shredded mozzarella cheese (medium-fat) – 3 cups

- Olive oil spray

- Onion (chopped) – 1 medium

- Spinach leaves – 8 ounces

- Half-and-half – 1 cup

- Black pepper – 1 teaspoon

- Feta cheese – 1/2 cup

Directions:

1. Begin by heating the oven to 375F.

2. Get a glass baking dish and grease it with olive oil spray. Arrange aside.

3. Now take a nonstick pan and pour in the olive oil. Position the pan on allows heat and allows it heat.

4. Immediately you are done, toss in the garlic, spinach, and onion. Prepare for about 5 minutes. Arrange aside.

5. You can now Get a large mixing bowl and add in the half, eggs, pepper, and salt. Whisk thoroughly to combine.

6. Put in the feta cheese and chopped mozzarella cheese (reserve 1/2 cup of mozzarella cheese for later).

7. Put the egg mixture and prepared spinach to the prepared glass baking dish. Blend well to combine. Drizzle the reserved cheese over the top.

8. Bake the egg mix for about 45 minutes.

9. Extract the baking dish from the oven and allow it to stand for 10 minutes.

10. Dice and serve!

Nutrition: Calories: 323 calories per serving Fat – 22.3 g Protein – 22.6 g Carbohydrates – 7.9 g

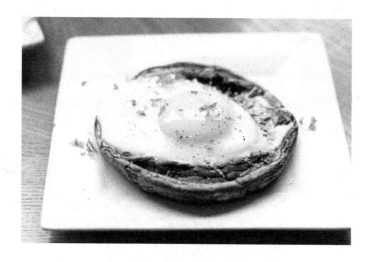

Quick Low-Carb Oatmeal

Preparation Time: 10 minutes

Cooking Time: 15 minutes

Servings: 2

Ingredients:

- Almond flour – 1/2 cup

- Flax meal – 2 tablespoons

- Cinnamon (ground) – 1 teaspoon

- Almond milk (unsweetened) – 11/2 cups

- Salt – as per taste

- Chia seeds – 2 tablespoons

- Liquid stevia – 10 – 15 drops

- Vanilla extract – 1 teaspoon

Directions:

1. Begin by taking a large mixing bowl and adding in the coconut flour, almond flour, ground cinnamon, flax seed powder, and chia seeds. Mix properly to combine.

2. Position a stockpot on a low heat and add in the dry ingredients. Also add in the liquid stevia, vanilla extract, and almond milk. Mix well to combine.

3. Prepare the flour and almond milk for about 4 minutes. Add salt if needed.

4. Move the oatmeal to a serving bowl and top with nuts, seeds, and pure and neat berries.

Nutrition: Calories: calories per serving Protein – 11.7 g Fat – 24.3 g Carbohydrates – 16.7 g

APPETIZER RECIPES

Alkaline Spring Salad

Preparation time: 10 minutes

Cooking time: 0 minutes

Servings: 1-2

Eating seasonal fruits and vegetables is a fabulous way of taking care of yourself and the environment at the same time. This alkaline-electric salad is delicious and nutritious.

Ingredients:

- 4 cups seasonal approved greens of your choice

- 1 cup cherry tomatoes

- 1/4 cup walnuts

- 1/4 cup approved herbs of your choice

- For the dressing:

- 3-4 key limes

- 1 tbsp. of homemade raw sesame

- Sea salt and cayenne pepper

Directions:

1. First, get the juice of the key limes. In a small bowl, whisk together the key lime juice with the homemade raw sesame "tahini" butter. Add sea salt and cayenne pepper, to taste.

2. Cut the cherry tomatoes in half.

3. In a large bowl, combine the greens, cherry tomatoes, and herbs. Pour the dressing on top and "massage" with your hands.

4. Let the greens soak up the dressing. Add more sea salt, cayenne pepper, and herbs on top if you wish. Enjoy!

Nutrition: Calories: 77 Carbohydrates: 11g

Fresh Tuna Salad

Preparation Time: 10 minutes

Cooking time: none

Servings: 3

Ingredients:

- 1 can tuna (6 oz.)

- 1/3 cup fresh cucumber, chopped

- 1/3 cup fresh tomato, chopped

- 1/3 cup avocado, chopped

- 1/3 cup celery, chopped

- 2 garlic cloves, minced

- 4 tsp. olive oil

- 2 tbsp. lime juice

- Pinch of black pepper

Directions:

1. Prepare the dressing by combining olive oil, lime juice, minced garlic and black pepper.

2. Mix the salad ingredients in a salad bowl and drizzle with the dressing.

Nutrition: Carbohydrates: 4.8 g Protein: 14.3 g Total sugars: 1.1 g Calories: 212 g

Roasted Portobello Salad

Preparation Time: 10 minutes

Cooking time: none

Servings: 4

Ingredients:

- 11/2 lb. Portobello mushrooms, stems trimmed

- 3 heads Belgian endive, sliced

- 1 small red onion, sliced

- 4 oz. blue cheese

- 8 oz. mixed salad greens

- Dressing:

- 3 tbsp. red wine vinegar

- 1 tbsp. Dijon mustard

- 2/3 cup olive oil

- Salt and pepper to taste

Directions:

1. Preheat the oven to 450F.

2. Prepare the dressing by whisking together vinegar, mustard, salt and pepper. Slowly add olive oil while whisking.

3. Cut the mushrooms and arrange them on a baking sheet, stem-side up. Coat the mushrooms with some dressing and bake for 15 minutes.

4. In a salad bowl toss the salad greens with onion, endive and cheese. Sprinkle with the dressing.

5. Add mushrooms to the salad bowl.

Nutrition: Carbohydrates: 22.3 g Protein: 14.9 g Total sugars: 2.1 g Calories: 501

Shredded Chicken Salad

Preparation Time: 5 minutes

Cooking time: 10 minutes

Servings: 6

Ingredients:

- 2 chicken breasts, boneless, skinless

- 1 head iceberg lettuce, cut into strips

- 2 bell peppers, cut into strips

- 1 fresh cucumber, quartered, sliced

- 3 scallions, sliced

- 2 tbsp. chopped peanuts

- 1 tbsp. peanut vinaigrette

- Salt to taste

- 1 cup water

Directions:

1. In a skillet simmer one cup of salted water.

2. Add the chicken breasts, cover and cook on low for 5 minutes. Remove the cover. Then remove the chicken from the skillet and shred with a fork.

3. In a salad bowl mix the vegetables with the cooled chicken, season with salt and sprinkle with peanut vinaigrette and chopped peanuts.

Nutrition: Carbohydrates: 9 g Protein: 11.6 g Total sugars: 4.2 g Calories: 117

Broccoli Salad

Preparation Time: 10 minutes

Cooking time: none

Servings: 6

Ingredients:

- 1 medium head broccoli, raw, florets only

- 1/2 cup red onion, chopped

- 12 oz. turkey bacon, chopped, fried until crisp

- 1/2 cup cherry tomatoes, halved

- ¼ cup sunflower kernels

- ¾ cup raisins

- ¾ cup mayonnaise

- 2 tbsp. white vinegar

Directions:

1. In a salad bowl combine the broccoli, tomatoes and onion.

2. Mix mayo with vinegar and sprinkle over the broccoli.

3. Add the sunflower kernels, raisins and bacon and toss well.

Nutrition: Carbohydrates: 17.3 g Protein: 11 g Total sugars: 10 g Calories: 220

FIRST COURSE RECIPES

Warm Barley and Squash Salad

Preparation Time: 20 minutes

Cooking Time: 40 minutes

Serving: 8

Ingredients:

- 1 small butternut squash

- 3 tablespoons extra-virgin olive oil

- 2 cups broccoli florets

- 1 cup pearl barley

- 1 cup toasted chopped walnuts

- 2 cups baby kale

- ½ red onion, sliced

- 2 tablespoons balsamic vinegar

- 2 garlic cloves, minced

- ½ teaspoon salt

- ¼ teaspoon black pepper

Direction:

1. Preheat the oven to 400°F. Line a baking sheet with parchment paper.

2. Peel off the squash, and slice into dice. In a large bowl, toss the squash with 2 teaspoons of olive oil. Transfer to the prepared baking sheet and roast for 20 minutes.

3. While the squash is roasting, toss the broccoli in the same bowl with 1 teaspoon of olive oil. After 20 minutes, flip the squash and push it to one side of the baking sheet. Add the broccoli to the other side and continue to roast for 20 more minutes until tender.

4. While the veggies are roasting, in a medium pot, cover the barley with several inches of water. Boil, then adjust heat, cover, and simmer for 30 minutes until tender. Drain and rinse.

5. Transfer the barley to a large bowl, and toss with the cooked squash and broccoli, walnuts, kale, and onion.

6. In a small bowl, mix the remaining 2 tablespoons of olive oil, balsamic vinegar, garlic, salt, and pepper. Drizzle dressing over the salad and toss.

Nutrition: 274 Calories 32g Carbohydrates 3g Sugars

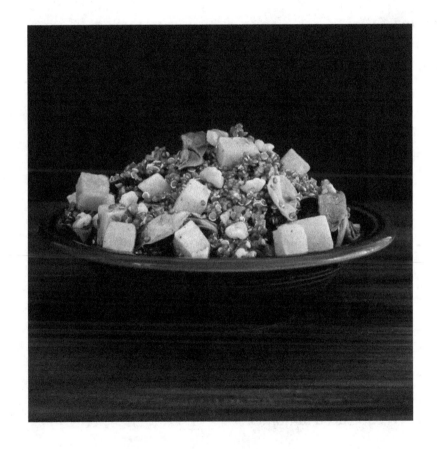

Winter Chicken and Citrus Salad

Preparation Time: 10 minutes

Cooking Time: 0 minute

Serving: 4

Ingredients:

- 4 cups baby spinach

- 2 tablespoons extra-virgin olive oil

- 1 tablespoon lemon juice

- 1/8 teaspoon salt

- 2 cups chopped cooked chicken

- 2 mandarin oranges

- ½ peeled grapefruit, sectioned

- ¼ cup sliced almonds

Direction:

1. Toss spinach with the olive oil, lemon juice, salt, and pepper.

2. Add the chicken, oranges, grapefruit, and almonds to the bowl. Toss gently.

3. Arrange on 4 plates and serve.

Nutrition: 249 Calories 11g Carbohydrates 7g Sugars

Pork Chops with Grape Sauce

Preparation Time: 15 minutes

Cooking Time: 25 minutes

Servings: 4

Ingredients:

- Cooking spray

- 4 pork chops

- ¼ cup onion, sliced

- 1 clove garlic, minced

- 1/2 cup low-sodium chicken broth

- ¾ cup apple juice

- 1 tablespoon cornstarch

- 1 tablespoon balsamic vinegar

- 1 teaspoon honey

- 1 cup seedless red grapes, sliced in half

Directions:

1. Spray oil on your pan.
2. Put it over medium heat.
3. Add the pork chops to the pan.
4. Cook for 5 minutes per side.
5. Remove and set aside.
6. Add onion and garlic.
7. Cook for 2 minutes.
8. Pour in the broth and apple juice.
9. Bring to a boil.
10. Reduce heat to simmer.
11. Put the pork chops back to the skillet.
12. Simmer for 4 minutes.
13. In a bowl, mix the cornstarch, vinegar and honey.
14. Add to the pan.
15. Cook until the sauce has thickened.
16. Add the grapes.
17. Pour sauce over the pork chops before serving.

Nutrition: Calories 188 Total Fat 4 g Saturated Fat 1 g Cholesterol 47 mg Sodium 117 mg Total Carbohydrate 18 g Dietary Fiber 1 g Total Sugars 13 g Protein 19 g Potassium 759 mg

SECOND COURSE RECIPES

Lemon Sole

Preparation Time: 10 minutes

Cooking Time: 5 Minutes

Servings: 2

Ingredients:

- 1lb sole fillets, boned and skinned

- 1 cup low sodium fish broth

- 2 shredded sweet onions

- juice of half a lemon

- 2tbsp dried cilantro

Directions:

1. Mix all the ingredients in your Instant Pot.

2. Cook on Stew for 5 minutes.

3. Release the pressure naturally.

Nutrition: Calories: 230; Carbs: Sugar: 1; Fat: 6; Protein: 46; GL: 1

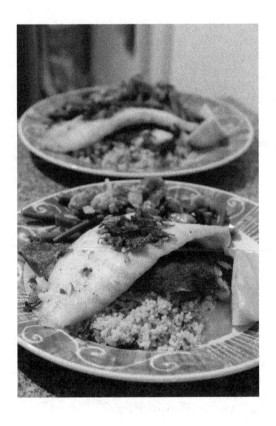

Tuna Sweet corn Casserole

Preparation Time: 10 minutes

Cooking Time: 35 Minutes

Servings: 2

Ingredients:

- 3 small tins of tuna

- 0.5lb sweet corn kernels

- 1lb chopped vegetables

- 1 cup low sodium vegetable broth

- 2tbsp spicy seasoning

Directions:

1. Mix all the ingredients in your Instant Pot.

2. Cook on Stew for 35 minutes.

3. Release the pressure naturally.

Nutrition: Calories: 300; Carbs: 6; Sugar: 1; Fat: 9; Protein: GL: 2

Lemon Pepper Salmon

Preparation Time: 10 minutes

Cooking Time: 10 Minutes

Servings: 4

Ingredients:

- 3 tbsps. ghee or avocado oil

- 1 lb. skin-on salmon filet

- 1 julienned red bell pepper

- 1 julienned green zucchini

- 1 julienned carrot

- ¾ cup water

- A few sprigs of parsley, tarragon, dill, basil or a combination

- 1/2 sliced lemon

- 1/2 tsp. black pepper

- ¼ tsp. sea salt

Directions:

1. Add the water and the herbs into the bottom of the Instant Pot and put in a wire steamer rack making sure the handles extend upwards.

2. Place the salmon filet onto the wire rack, with the skin side facing down.

3. Drizzle the salmon with ghee, season with black pepper and salt, and top with the lemon slices.

4. Close and seal the Instant Pot, making sure the vent is turned to "Sealing".

5. Select the "Steam" setting and cook for 3 minutes.

6. While the salmon cooks, julienne the vegetables, and set aside.

7. Once done, quick release the pressure, and then press the "Keep Warm/Cancel" button.

8. Uncover and wearing oven mitts, carefully remove the steamer rack with the salmon.

9. Remove the herbs and discard them.

10. Add the vegetables to the pot and put the lid back on.

11. Select the "Sauté" function and cook for 1-2 minutes.

12. Serve the vegetables with salmon and add the remaining fat to the pot.

13. Pour a little of the sauce over the fish and vegetables if desired.

Nutrition: Calories 296, Carbs 8g, Fat 15 g, Protein 31 g, Potassium (K) 1084 mg, Sodium (Na) 284 mg

Baked Salmon with Garlic Parmesan Topping

Preparation time: 5 minutes,

Cooking time: 20 minutes,

Servings: 4

Ingredients:

- 1 lb. wild caught salmon filets

- 2 tbsp. margarine

- What you'll need from store cupboard:

- ¼ cup reduced fat parmesan cheese, grated

- ¼ cup light mayonnaise

- 2-3 cloves garlic, diced

- 2 tbsp. parsley

- Salt and pepper

Directions:

1. Heat oven to 350 and line a baking pan with parchment paper.

2. Place salmon on pan and season with salt and pepper.

3. In a medium skillet, over medium heat, melt butter. Add garlic and cook, stirring 1 minute.

4. Reduce heat to low and add remaining Ingredients. Stir until everything is melted and combined.

5. Spread evenly over salmon and bake 15 minutes for thawed fish or 20 for frozen. Salmon is done when it flakes easily with a fork. Serve.

Nutrition: Calories 408 Total Carbs 4g Protein 41g Fat 24g Sugar 1g Fiber 0g

Blackened Shrimp

Preparation time: 5 minutes

Cooking time: 5 minutes

Servings: 4

Ingredients:

- 1 1/2 lbs. shrimp, peel & devein

- 4 lime wedges

- 4 tbsp. cilantro, chopped

- What you'll need from store cupboard:

- 4 cloves garlic, diced

- 1 tbsp. chili powder

- 1 tbsp. paprika

- 1 tbsp. olive oil

- 2 tsp. Splenda brown sugar

- 1 tsp. cumin

- 1 tsp. oregano

- 1 tsp. garlic powder

- 1 tsp. salt

- 1/2 tsp. pepper

Directions:

1. In a small bowl combine seasonings and Splenda brown sugar.

2. Heat oil in a skillet over med-high heat. Add shrimp, in a single layer, and cook 1-2 minutes per side.

3. Add seasonings, and cook, stirring, 30 seconds. Serve garnished with cilantro and a lime wedge.

Nutrition: Calories 252 Total Carbs 7g Net Carbs 6g Protein 39g Fat 7g Sugar 2g Fiber 1g

SIDE DISH RECIPES

Zucchini Pepper Chips

Preparation time: 10 minutes

Cooking time: 15 minutes

Servings: 04

Ingredients:

- 1 2/3 cups vegetable oil

- 1 teaspoon garlic powder

- 1 teaspoon onion powder

- 1/2 teaspoon black pepper

- 3 tablespoons crushed red pepper flakes

- 2 zucchinis, thinly sliced

Directions:

1. Mix oil with all the spices in a bowl.

2. Add zucchini slices and mix well.

3. Transfer the mixture to a Ziplock bag and seal it.

4. Refrigerate for 10 minutes.

5. Spread the zucchini slices on a greased baking sheet.

6. Bake for 15 minutes

7. Serve.

Nutrition: Calories 172 Total Fat 11.1 g Saturated Fat 5.8 g Cholesterol 610 mg Sodium 749 mgTotal Carbs 19.9 g Fiber 0.2 g Sugar 0.2 g Protein 13.5 g

Apple Chips

Preparation time: 5 minutes

Cooking time: 45 minutes

Servings:4

Ingredients:

- 2 Golden Delicious apples, cored and thinly sliced

- 1 1/2 teaspoons white sugar

- 1/2 teaspoon ground cinnamon

Directions:

1. Set your oven to 225 degrees F.

2. Place apple slices on a baking sheet.

3. Sprinkle sugar an

4. d cinnamon over apple slices.

5. Bake for 45 minutes.

6. Serve

Nutrition: Calories 127 Total Fat 3.5 g Saturated Fat 0.5 g Cholesterol 162 mg Sodium 142 mg Total Carbs 33.6g Fiber 0.4 g Sugar 0.5 g Protein 4.5 g

Kale Crisps

Preparation time: 10 minutes

Cooking time: 10 minutes

Servings: 04

Ingredients:

- 1 bunch kale, remove the stems, leaves torn into even pieces

- 1 tablespoon olive oil

- 1 teaspoon sea salt

Directions:

1. Set your oven to 350 degrees F. Layer a baking sheet with parchment paper.

2. Spread the kale leaves on a paper towel to absorb all the moisture.

3. Toss the leaves with sea salt, and olive oil.

4. Kindly spread them, on the baking sheet and bake for 10 minutes.

5. Serve.

Nutrition: Calories 113 Total Fat 7.5 g Saturated Fat 1.1 g Cholesterol 20 mg Sodium 97 mg Total Carbs 1.4 g Fiber 0 g Sugar 0 g Protein 1.1g

SOUP & STEW

Cream of Tomato Soup

Preparation time: 15 minutes

Cooking time: 15 minutes

Servings: 2

Ingredients:

- 1lb fresh tomatoes, chopped

- 1.5 cups low sodium tomato puree

- 1tbsp black pepper

Directions:

1. Mix all the ingredients in your Instant Pot.

2. Cook on Stew for 15 minutes.

3. Release the pressure naturally.

4. Blend.

Nutrition: Calories: 20 Carbs: 2 Sugar: 1 Fat: 0 Protein: 3 GL: 1

Shiitake Soup

Preparation time: 15 minutes

Cooking time: 35 minutes

Servings: 2

Ingredients:

- 1 cup shiitake mushrooms

- 1 cup diced vegetables

- 1 cup low sodium vegetable broth

- 2tbsp 5 spice seasoning

Directions:

1. Mix all the ingredients in your Instant Pot.

2. Cook on Stew for 35 minutes.

3. Release the pressure naturally.

Nutrition: Calories: 70 Carbs: 5 Sugar: 1 Fat: 2 Protein: 2 GL: 1

Spicy Pepper Soup

Preparation time: 15 minutes

Cooking time: 15 minutes

Servings: 2

Ingredients:

- 1lb chopped mixed sweet peppers

- 1 cup low sodium vegetable broth

- 3tbsp chopped chili peppers

- 1tbsp black pepper

Directions:

1. Mix all the ingredients in your Instant Pot.

2. Cook on Stew for 15 minutes.

3. Release the pressure naturally. Blend.

Nutrition: Calories: 100 Carbs: 11 Sugar: 4 Fat: 2 Protein: 3 GL: 6

Zoodle Won-Ton Soup

Preparation time: 15 minutes

Cooking time: 5 minutes

Servings: 2

Ingredients:

- 1lb spiralized zucchini

- 1 pack unfried won-tons

- 1 cup low sodium beef broth

- 2tbsp soy sauce

Directions:

1. Mix all the ingredients in your Instant Pot.

2. Cook on Stew for 5 minutes.

3. Release the pressure naturally.

Nutrition: Calories: 300 Carbs: 6 Sugar: 1 Fat: 9 Protein: 43 GL: 2

Broccoli Stilton Soup

Preparation time: 15 minutes

Cooking time: 35 minutes

Servings: 2

Ingredients:

- 1lb chopped broccoli

- 0.5lb chopped vegetables

- 1 cup low sodium vegetable broth

- 1 cup Stilton

Directions:

1. Mix all the ingredients in your Instant Pot.

2. Cook on Stew for 35 minutes.

3. Release the pressure naturally.

4. Blend the soup.

Nutrition: Calories: 280 Carbs: 9 Sugar: 2 Fat: 22 Protein: 13 GL: 4

DESSERT

Chia Vanilla Coconut Pudding

Preparation time: 5 minutes

Cooking time: 5 minutes

Servings: 2

Ingredients:

- Coconut oil, 2 tablespoons

- Raw cashew, ½ cup

- Coconut water, ½ cup

- Cinnamon, 1 teaspoon

- Dates (pitted), 3

- Vanilla, 2 teaspoons

- Coconut flakes (unsweetened), 1 teaspoon

- Salt (Himalayan or Celtic Grey)

- Chia seeds, 6 tablespoons

- Cinnamon or pomegranate seeds for garnish (optional)

Directions:

1. Get a blender, add all the **Ingredients** (minus the pomegranate and chia seeds), and blend for about forty to sixty seconds.

2. Reduce the blender speed to the lowest and add the chia seeds.

3. Pour the content into an airtight container and put in a refrigerator for five to six hours.

4. To serve, you can garnish with the cinnamon powder of pomegranate seeds.

Nutrition: Calories: 201 Fat: 10 g Sodium: 32.8 mg

Sweet Tahini Dip with Ginger Cinnamon Fruit

Preparation time: 10 minutes

Cooking time: 5 minutes

Servings: 2

Ingredients:

- Cinnamon, one (1) teaspoon

- Green apple, one (1)

- Pear, one (1)

- Fresh ginger, two (2) – three (3)

- Celtic sea salt, one (1) teaspoon

- Ingredient for sweet Tahini

- Almond butter (raw), three (3) teaspoons

- Tahini (one big scoop), three (3) teaspoons

- Coconut oil, two (2) teaspoons

- Cayenne (optional), ¼ teaspoons

- Wheat-free tamari, two (2) teaspoons

- Liquid coconut nectar, one (1) teaspoon

Directions:

1. Get a clean mixing bowl.

2. Grate the ginger, add cinnamon, sea salt and mix together in the bowl.

3. Dice apple and pear into little cubes, turn into the bowl and mix.

4. Get a mixing bowl and mix all the **Ingredients**.

5. Then add the Sprinkle the Sweet Tahini Dip all over the Ginger Cinnamon Fruit.

6. Serve.

Nutrition: Calories: 109 Fat: 10.8 g Sodium: 258 mg

Coconut Butter and Chopped Berries with Mint

Preparation time: 5 minutes

Cooking time: 5 minutes

Servings: 04

Ingredients:

- Chopped mint, one (1) tablespoon

- Coconut butter (melted), two (2) tablespoons

- Mixed berries (strawberries, blueberries, and raspberries)

Directions:

1. Get a small bowl and add the berries.

2. Drizzle the melted coconut butter and sprinkle the mint.

3. Serve.

Nutrition: Calories: 159 Fat: 12 g Carbohydrates: 18 g

Alkaline Raw Pumpkin Pie

Preparation time: 5 minutes

Cooking time: 5 minutes

Servings: 04

Ingredients:

Ingredients for Pie Crust

- Cinnamon, one (1) teaspoon

- Dates/Turkish apricots, one (1) cup

- Raw almonds, one (1) cup

- Coconut flakes (unsweetened), one (1) cup

Ingredients for Pie Filling

- Dates, six (6)

- Cinnamon, ½ teaspoon

- Nutmeg, ½ teaspoon

- Pecans (soaked overnight), one (1) cup

- Organic pumpkin Blends (12 oz.), 1 ¼ cup

- Nutmeg, ½ teaspoon

- Sea salt (Himalayan or Celtic Sea Salt), ¼ teaspoon

- Vanilla, 1 teaspoon

- Gluten-free tamari

Directions:

Directions for pie crust

1. Get a food processor and blend all the pie crust **Ingredients** at the same time.

2. Make sure the mixture turns oily and sticky before you stop mixing.

3. Put the mixture in a pie pan and mold against the sides and floor, to make it stick properly.

Directions for the pie filling

1. Mix Ingredients together in a blender.

2. Add the mixture to fill in the pie crust.

3. Pour some cinnamon on top.

4. Then refrigerate till it's cold.

5. Then mold.

Nutrition: Calories 135 Calories from Fat 41.4.Total Fat 4.6 g
Cholesterol 11.3 mg

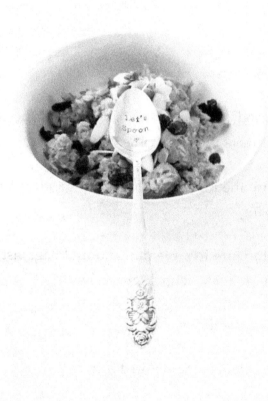

Strawberry Sorbet

Preparation time: 5 minutes

Cooking time: 4 Hours

Servings: 4

Ingredients:

- 2 cups of Strawberries*

- 1 1/2 teaspoons of Spelt Flour

- 1/2 cup of Date Sugar

- 2 cups of Spring Water

Directions:

- Add Date Sugar, Spring Water, and Spelt Flour to a medium pot and boil on low heat for about ten minutes. Mixture should thicken, like syrup.

- Remove the pot from the heat and allow it to cool.

- After cooling, add Blend Strawberry and mix gently.

- Put mixture in a container and freeze.

- Cut it into pieces, put the sorbet into a processor and blend until smooth.

- Put everything back in the container and leave in the refrigerator for at least four hours.

- Serve and enjoy your Strawberry Sorbet!

Nutrition: Calories: 198 Carbohydrates: 28 g

Blueberry Muffins

Preparation time: 5 minutes

Cooking time: 1 Hour

Servings: 3

Ingredients:

- 1/2 cup of Blueberries

- 3/4 cup of Teff Flour

- 3/4 cup of Spelt Flour

- 1/3 cup of Agave Syrup

- 1/2 teaspoon of Pure Sea Salt

- 1 cup of Coconut Milk

- 1/4 cup of Sea Moss Gel (optional, check information)

- Grape Seed Oil

Directions:

1. Preheat your oven to 365 degrees Fahrenheit.

2. Grease or line 6 standard muffin cups.

3. Add Teff, Spelt flour, Pure Sea Salt, Coconut Milk, Sea Moss Gel, and Agave Syrup to a large bowl. Mix them together.

4. Add Blueberries to the mixture and mix well.

5. Divide muffin batter among the 6 muffin cups.

6. Bake for 30 minutes until golden brown.

7. Serve and enjoy your Blueberry Muffins!

Nutrition: Calories: 65 Fat: 0.7 g Carbohydrates: 12 g Protein: 1.4 g Fiber: 5 g

Banana Strawberry Ice Cream

Preparation time: 5 minutes

Cooking time: 4 Hours

Servings: 5

Ingredients:

- 1 cup of Strawberry*

- 5 quartered Baby Bananas*

- 1/2 Avocado, chopped

- 1 tablespoon of Agave Syrup

- 1/4 cup of Homemade Walnut Milk

Directions:

1. Mix Ingredients into the blender and blend them well.

2. Taste. If it is too thick, add extra Milk or Agave Syrup if you want it sweeter.

3. Put in a container with a lid and allow to freeze for at least 5 to 6 hours.

4. Serve it and enjoy your Banana Strawberry Ice Cream!

Nutrition: Calories: 200 Fat: 0.5 g Carbohydrates: 44 g

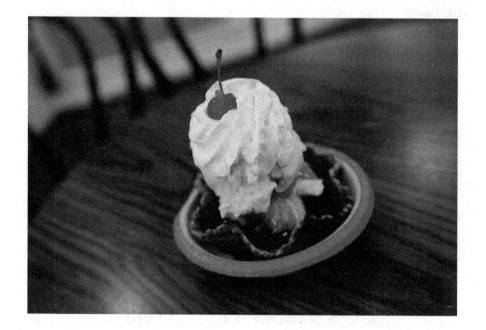

Homemade Whipped Cream

Preparation time: 5 minutes

Cooking time: 10 Minutes

Servings: 1 Cup

Ingredients:

- 1 cup of Aquafaba

- 1/4 cup of Agave Syrup

Directions:

1. Add Agave Syrup and Aquafaba into a bowl.

2. Mix at high speed around 5 minutes with a stand mixer or 10 to 15 minutes with a hand mixer.

3. Serve and enjoy your Homemade Whipped Cream!

Nutrition: Calories: 21 Fat: 0g Sodium: 0.3g Carbohydrates: 5.3g Fiber: 0g Sugars: 4.7g Protein: 0g

JUICE AND SMOOTHIE RECIPES

Apple – Banana Smoothie (Abs)

Preparation time: 10 minutes

Cooking time: 0 minutes

Servings: 1

Ingredients:

- I Cup Cubed Apple

- ½ Burro Banana

- ½ Cup Cubed Mango

- ½ Cup Cubed Watermelon

- ½ Teaspoon Powdered Onion

- 3 Tablespoon Key Lime Juice

- Date Sugar to Taste (If you like)

Directions:

1. In a clean bowl rinse, the vegetable with clean water.

2. Cubed Banana, Apple, Mango, Watermelon and add other items into the blender and blend to achieve homogenous smoothies.

3. Serve your delicious medicinal detox.

4. Alternatively, you can add one tablespoon of finely dices raw red Onion if powdered Onion is not available.

Nutrition: Calories: 99 Fat: 0.3g Carbohydrates: 23 grams Protein: 1.1 g

Ginger – Pear Smoothie (GPS)

Preparation time: 10 minutes

Cooking time: 0 minutes

Servings: 1

Ingredients:

- 1 Big Pear with Seed and Cured

- ½ Avocado

- ¼ Handful Watercress

- ½ Sour Orange

- ½ Cup Ginger Tea

- ½ Cup Coconut Water

- ¼ Cup Spring Water

- 2 Tablespoon Agave Syrup

- Date Sugar to satisfaction

Directions:

1. Firstly boil 1 cup of Ginger Tea, cover the cup and allow it cool to room temperature.

2. Pour all the AGPS Items into your clean blender and homogenize them to smooth fluid.

3. You have just prepared yourself a wonderful Detox Romaine Smoothie.

Nutrition: Calories: 101. Protein: 1 g Carbs: 27 g Fiber: 6 g

Cantaloupe – Amaranth Smoothie (CAS)

Preparation time: 10 minutes

Cooking time: 0 minutes

Servings: 1

Ingredients:

- ½ Cup Cubed Cantaloupe

- ¼ Handful Green Amaranth

- ½ Cup Homemade Hemp Milk

- ¼ Teaspoon Dr. Sebi's Bromide Plus Powder

- 1 Cup Coconut Water

- 1 Teaspoon Agave Syrup

Directions:

1. You will have to rinse all the ACAS items with clean water.

2. Chop green Amaranth, cubed Cantaloupe, transfer all into a blender and blend to achieve homogenous smoothie.

3. Pour into a clean cup; add Agave syrup and homemade Hemp Milk.

4. Stir them together and drink.

Nutrition: Calories: 55 Fiber: 1.5 g Carbohydrates: 8 mg

Garbanzo Squash Smoothie (GSS)

Preparation time: 10 minutes

Cooking time: 0 minutes

Servings: 1

Ingredients:

- 1 Large Cubed Apple

- 1 Fresh Tomatoes

- 1 Tablespoon Finely Chopped Fresh Onion or ¼ Teaspoon Powdered Onion

- ¼ Cup Boiled Garbanzo Bean

- ½ Cup Coconut Milk

- ¼ Cubed Mexican Squash Chayote

- 1 Cup Energy Booster Tea

Directions:

1. You will need to rinse the AGSS items with clean water.

2. Boil 1½ Dr. Sebi's Energy Booster Tea with 2 cups of clean water. Filter the extract, measure 1 cup and allow it to cool.

3. Cook Garbanzo Bean, drain the water and allow it to cool.

4. Pour all the AGSS items into a high-speed blender and blend to achieve homogenous smoothie.

5. You may add Date Sugar.

6. Serve your amazing smoothie and drink.

Nutrition: Calories: 82. Carbs: 22 g Protein: 2 g Fiber: 7 g

Strawberry – Orange Smoothies (SOS)

Preparation time: 10 minutes

Cooking time: 0 minutes

Servings: 1

Ingredients:

- 1 Cup Diced Strawberries

- 1 Removed Back of Seville Orange

- ¼ Cup Cubed Cucumber

- ¼ Cup Romaine Lettuce

- ½ Kelp

- ½ Burro Banana

- 1 Cup Soft Jelly Coconut Water

- ½ Cup Water

- Date Sugar.

Directions:

1. Use clean water to rinse all the vegetable items of ASOS into a clean bowl.

2. Chop Romaine Lettuce; dice Strawberry, Cucumber, and Banana; remove the back of Seville Orange and divide into four.

3. Transfer all the ASOS items inside a clean blender and blend to achieve a homogenous smoothie.

4. Pour into a clean big cup and fortify your body with a palatable detox.

Nutrition: Calories 298 Calories from Fat 9.Fat 1g Cholesterol 2mg Sodium 73mg Potassium 998mg

Carbohydrates 68g Fiber 7g Sugar 50g

Tamarind – Pear Smoothie (TPS)

Preparation time: 10 minutes

Cooking time: 0 minutes

Servings: 1

Ingredients:

- ½ Burro Banana

- ½ Cup Watermelon

- 1 Raspberries

- 1 Prickly Pear

- 1 Grape with Seed

- 3 Tamarind

- ½ Medium Cucumber

- 1 Cup Coconut Water

- ½ Cup Distilled Water

Directions:

1. Use clean water to rinse all the ATPS items.

2. Remove the pod of Tamarind and collect the edible part around the seed into a container.

3. If you must use the seeds then you have to boil the seed for 15mins and add to the Tamarind edible part in the container.

4. Cubed all other vegetable fruits and transfer all the items into a high-speed blender and blend to achieve homogenous smoothie.

Nutrition: Calories: 199 Carbohydrates: 47 g Fat: 1g Protein: 6g

Currant Elderberry Smoothie (CES)

Preparation time: 10 minutes

Cooking time: 0 minutes

Servings: 1

Ingredients:

- ¼ Cup Cubed Elderberry

- 1 Sour Cherry

- 2 Currant

- 1 Cubed Burro Banana

- 1 Fig

- 1Cup 4 Bay Leaves Tea

- 1 Cup Energy Booster Tea

- Date Sugar to your satisfaction

Directions:

1. Use clean water to rinse all the ACES items

2. Initially boil ¾ Teaspoon of Energy Booster Tea with 2 cups of water on a heat source and allow boiling for 10 minutes.

3. Add 4 Bay leaves and boil together for another 4minutes.

4. Drain the Tea extract into a clean big cup and allow it to cool.

5. Transfer all the items into a high-speed blender and blend till you achieve a homogenous smoothie.

6. Pour the palatable medicinal smoothie into a clean cup and drink.

Nutrition: Calories: 63 Fat: 0.22g Sodium: 1.1mg Carbohydrates: 15.5g Fiber: 4.8g Sugars: 8.25g Protein: 1.6g

Sweet Dream Strawberry Smoothie

Preparation time:1 5 minutes

Cooking time: 0

Servings: 1

Ingredients:

- 5 Strawberries

- 3 Dates – Pits eliminated

- 2 Burro Bananas or small bananas

- Spring Water for 32 fluid ounces of smoothie

Directions:

1. Strip off skin of the bananas.

2. Wash the dates and strawberries.

3. Include bananas, dates, and strawberries to a blender container.

4. Include a couple of water and blend.

5. Keep on including adequate water to persuade up to be 32 oz. of smoothie.

Nutrition: Calories: 282 Fat: 11g Carbohydrates: 4g Protein: 7g

Alkaline Green Ginger and Banana Cleansing Smoothie

Preparation time: 15 minutes

Cooking time: 0

Servings: 1

Ingredients:

- One handful of kale

- one banana, frozen

- Two cups of hemp seed milk

- One inch of ginger, finely minced

- Half cup of chopped strawberries, frozen

- 1 tablespoon of agave or your preferred sweetener

Directions:

1. Mix all the **Ingredients** in a blender and mix on high speed.

2. Allow it to blend evenly.

3. Pour into a pitcher with a few decorative straws and voila you are one happy camper.

4. Enjoy!

Nutrition: Calories: 350 Fat: 4g Carbohydrates: 52g Protein: 16g

Orange Mixed Detox Smoothie

Preparation time: 15 minutes

Cooking time: 0

Servings: 1

Ingredients:

- One cup of vegies (Amaranth, Dandelion, Lettuce or Watercress)

- Half avocado

- One cup of tender-jelly coconut water

- One seville orange

- Juice of one key lime

- One tablespoon of bromide plus powder

Directions:

1. Peel and cut the Seville orange in chunks.

2. Mix all the **Ingredients** collectively in a high-speed blender until done.

Nutrition: Calories: 71 Fat: 1g Carbohydrates: 12g Protein: 2g

Cucumber Toxin Flush Smoothie

Preparation time: 15 minutes

Cooking time: 0

Servings: 1

Ingredients:

- 1 Cucumber

- 1 Key Lime

- 1 cup of watermelon (seeded), cubed

Directions:

1. Mix all the above **Ingredients** in a high-speed blender.

2. Considering that watermelon and cucumbers are largely water, you may not want to add any extra, however you can so if you want.

3. Juice the key lime and add into your smoothie.

4. Enjoy!

Nutrition: Calories: 219 Fat: 4g Carbohydrates: 48g Protein: 5g

OTHER DIABETIC RECIPES

Dairy-Free Fruit Tarts

Preparation time: 15 minutes

Cooking time: 15 minutes

Servings: 2

Ingredients:

- 1 cup Coconut Whipped Cream
- ½ Easy Shortbread Crust (dairy-free option)
- Fresh mint Sprigs
- ½ cup mixed fresh Berries

Directions:

1. Grease two 4″ pans with detachable bottoms. Pour the shortbread mixture into pans and firmly press into the edges and bottom of each pan. Refrigerate for 15 minutes.
2. Loosen the crust carefully to remove from the pan.
3. Distribute the whipped cream between the tarts and evenly spread to the sides. Refrigerate for 1-2 hours to make it firm.

4. Use the berries and sprig of mint to garnish each of the tarts

Nutrition: Fat: 28.9g Carbs: 8.3g Protein: 5.8g Calories: 306

Spaghetti Squash with Peanut Sauce

Preparation time: 15 minutes

Cooking time: 15 minutes

Servings: 4

Ingredients:

- 1 cup cooked shelled edamame; frozen, thawed

- 3-pound spaghetti squash

- ½ cup red bell pepper, sliced

- ¼ cup scallions, sliced

- 1 medium carrot, shredded

- 1 teaspoon minced garlic

- ½ teaspoon crushed red pepper

- 1 tablespoon rice vinegar

- ¼ cup coconut aminos

- 1 tablespoon maple syrup

- ½ cup peanut butter

- ¼ cup unsalted roasted peanuts, chopped

- ¼ cup and 2 tablespoons spring water, divided

- ¼ cup fresh cilantro, chopped

- 4 lime wedges

Directions:

1. Prepare the squash: cut each squash in half lengthwise and then remove seeds.

2. Take a microwave-proof dish, place squash halves in it cut-side-up, drizzle with 2 tablespoons water, and then microwave at high heat setting for 10–15 minutes until tender.

3. Let squash cool for 15 minutes until able to handle. Use a fork to scrape its flesh lengthwise to make noodles, and then let noodles cool for 10 minutes.

4. While squash microwaves, prepare the sauce: take a medium bowl, add butter in it along with red pepper and garlic, pour in vinegar, coconut aminos, maple syrup, and water, and then whisk until smooth.

5. When the squash noodles have cooled, distribute them evenly among four bowls, top with scallions, carrots, bell pepper, and edamame beans, and then drizzle with prepared sauce.

6. Sprinkle cilantro and peanuts and serve each bowl with a lime wedge.

Nutrition: Calories: 419 Carbohydrates: 32.8 grams Fat: 24 grams Protein: 17.6 grams

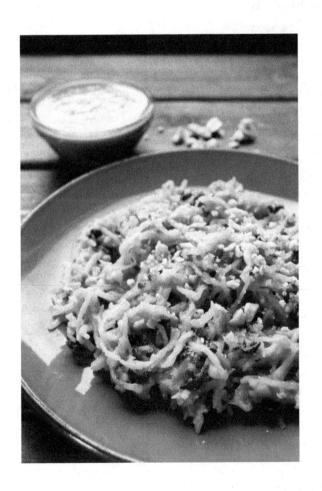

Cauliflower Alfredo Pasta

Preparation time: 10 minutes

Cooking time: 30 minutes

Servings: 4

Ingredients:

- Alfredo sauce

- 4 cups cauliflower florets, fresh

- 1 tablespoon minced garlic

- ¼ cup **Nutrition**al yeast

- ½ teaspoon garlic powder

- ¾ teaspoon sea salt

- ½ teaspoon onion powder

- ½ teaspoon ground black pepper

- ½ tablespoon olive oil

- 1 tablespoon lemon juice, and more as needed for serving

- ½ cup almond milk, unsweetened

- Pasta

- 1 tablespoon minced parsley

- 1 lemon, juiced

- ½ teaspoon sea salt

- ¼ teaspoon ground black pepper

- 12 ounces spelt pasta; cooked, warmed

Directions:

1. Take a large pot half full with water, place it over medium-high heat, and then bring it to a boil.

2. Add cauliflower florets, cook for 10–15 minutes until tender, drain them well, and then return florets to the pot.

3. Take a medium skillet pan, place it over low heat, add oil and when hot, add garlic and cook for 4–5 minutes until fragrant and golden-brown.

4. Spoon garlic into a food processor, add remaining **Ingredients** for the sauce in it, along with cauliflower florets, and then pulse for 2–3 minutes until smooth.

5. Tip the sauce into the pot, stir it well, place it over medium-low heat, and then cook for 5 minutes until hot.

6. Add pasta into the pot, toss well until coated, taste to adjust seasoning, and then cook for 2 minutes until pasta gets hot.

7. Divide pasta and sauce among four plates, season with salt and black pepper, drizzle with lemon juice, and then top with minced parsley.

8. Serve straight away.

Nutrition: Calories: 360 Carbohydrates: 59 grams Fat: 9 grams Protein: 13 grams

Sloppy Joe

Preparation time: 8 minutes

Cooking time: 12 minutes

Servings: 4

Ingredients:

- 2 cups kamut or spelt wheat, cooked

- ½ cup white onion, diced

- 1 roma tomato, diced

- 1 cup chickpeas, cooked

- ½ cup green bell peppers, diced

- 1 teaspoon sea salt

- 1/8 teaspoon cayenne pepper

- 1 teaspoon onion powder

- 1 tablespoon grapeseed oil

- 1 ½ cups barbecue sauce, alkaline

Directions:

1. Plug in a high-power food processor, add chickpeas and spelt, cover with the lid, and then pulse for 15 seconds.

2. Take a large skillet pan, place it over medium-high heat, add oil and when hot, add onion and bell pepper, season with salt, cayenne pepper, and onion powder, and then stir until well combined.

3. Cook the vegetables for 3–5 minutes until tender. Add tomatoes, add the pulsed mixture, pour in barbecue sauce, and then stir until well mixed.

4. Simmer for 5 minutes, then remove the pan from heat and serve sloppy joe with alkaline flatbread.

Nutrition: Calories: 333 Carbohydrates: 65 grams Fat: 5 grams Protein: 14 grams

Amaretti

Preparation time: 15 minutes

Cooking time: 22 minutes

Servings: 2

Ingredients:

- ½ cup of granulated Erythritol-based Sweetener

- 165g (2 cups) sliced Almonds

- ¼ cup of powdered of Erythritol-based sweetener

- 4 large egg whites

- Pinch of salt

- ½ tsp. almond extract

Directions:

1. Heat the oven to 300° F and use parchment paper to line 2 baking sheets. Grease the parchment slightly.
2. Process the powdered sweetener, granulated sweetener, and sliced almonds in a food processor until it appears like coarse crumbs.
3. Beat the egg whites plus the salt and almond extracts using an electric mixer in a large bowl until they hold

soft peaks. Fold in the almond mixture so that it becomes well combined.

4. Drop spoonful of the dough onto the prepared baking sheet and allow for a space of 1 inch between them. Press a sliced almond into the top of each cookie.

5. Bake in the oven for 22 minutes until the sides becomes brown. They will appear jellylike when they are taken out from the oven but will begin to be firms as it cools down.

Nutrition: Fat: 8.8g Carbs: 4.1g Protein: 5.3g Calories: 117

Green Fruit Juice

Preparation time: 10 minutes

Cooking time: 0 minutes

Servings: 2

Ingredients:

- 3 large kiwis, peeled and chopped

- 3 large green apples, cored and sliced

- 2 cups seedless green grapes

- 2 teaspoons fresh lime juice

Directions:

1. Add all ingredients into a juicer and extract the juice according to the manufacturer's method.
2. Pour into 2 glasses and serve immediately.

Nutrition: Calories 304 Total Fat 2.2 g Saturated Fat 0 g Protein 6.2 g

Kale Chickpea Mash

Preparation time: 15 minutes

Cooking time: 12 minutes

Servings: 1

Ingredients:

- 1 shallot

- 3 tbsp garlic

- A bunch of kale

- 1/2 cup boiled chickpea

- 2 tbsp coconut oil

- Sea salt

Directions:

1. Add some garlic in olive oil

2. Chop shallot and fry it with oil in a nonstick skillet.

3. Cook until the shallot turns golden brown.

4. Add kale and garlic in the skillet and stir well.

5. Add chickpeas and cook for 6 minutes. Add the rest of the **Ingredients** and give a good stir.

6. Serve and enjoy

Nutrition: Calories: 149 Total fat: 8 grams Saturated fat: 1 gram Net carbohydrates: 13 grams Protein: 4 grams Sugars 6g Fiber 3g Sodium 226mg Potassium 205mg

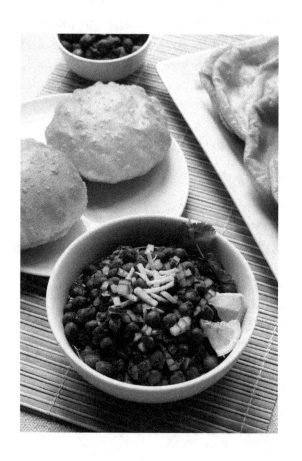